Heal-thy LiFE™

Heal-thy Land

2nd Edition

DR. CAROLYN G. ANDERSON

Heal-thy LiFE™

Heal-thy Land

2nd Edition

Copyright © 2017 by Dr. Carolyn G. Anderson

Published & Designed by Riley Press
A Division of Integrity Production & Publication
Chicago, Illinois
www.RileyPress.com

Printed in the United States of America.

All scripture references are noted and were either taken from the NIV, MSG, KJV or AMP versions of the Bible. Other references were noted within the text and will not have its own reference page.

ISBN-13: 978-0996403832
ISBN-10: 0996403833

Table of Contents

Dedication

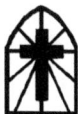

This book is dedicated to YOU, your Health, your Healing and the Healing of the Land!

Join the Book Club Group on Facebook and stay connected with us!

DrCarolynBookClub

Preface

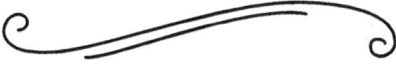

Have you ever had a dream that was so great that you wish that it was real and you were disappointed to wake up out of it? Or have you ever had those dreams that were more like nightmares and you were thrilled when you woke up and realized that it was just a dream? Well, life is sometimes like the good and the not so good dreams.

There are moments where everything seems great and all is going well and then there are those moments where it seems like an unending nightmare. This unending nightmare can be a desperate need for healing in your body, finance, your faith or relationships. Dealing with any unhealthy area of life can be compared to a nightmare; whether it's a physical, mental, or a spiritual matter.

One of the most lethal nightmare is the emotional pain that comes from a broken relationship or a broken heart and it's time to be free from the pain that you may have been carrying.

Life's not so good nightmares or dreams can enter your life during childhood years and oftentimes they go un-resolved. Well, now is the time to tackle those buried, un-resolved issues head-on and experience the joy that comes with living a whole carefree life.

There are so many facets of life that can leave unhealthy residues and leave one feeling like it's an all-day dream that's not ending and that is being in debt or having financial difficulties. On one end, you need finances to take care of your health, and on the other hand, financial problems can cause unhealthy stressors. Regardless of the type of unhealthy issue that you may be facing, it's my hope that this book will bring you one step closer towards living a healthy life.

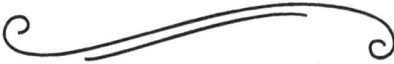

Introduction

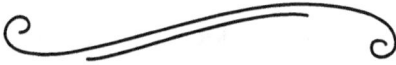

The first place that healing appears in the Bible is in the book Genesis. According to Genesis 20:17 AMP, "So Abraham prayed to God, and God healed Abimelech and his wife and his female slaves, and they bore children," and the NIV version says, "Then Abraham prayed to God, and God healed Abimelek, his wife and his female slaves so they could have children again." So, the very first healing ever in the history of mankind was performed by God himself through the prayer of Abraham.

As you read the 20th Chapter of Genesis, it's rather interesting that the healing that was needed was to open the womb of the king's wife and the females in his midst so that they could reproduce. The ability to not reproduce is death to a family and death to the land. Without the ability to reproduce, life would become extinct and creation would be non-existent. The king was in desperate need for healing as he didn't want to see his destiny and lineage come to a haul.

The same is true for you. Don't allow an un-healthy situation to cause you to leave your legacy prematurely. Pray and ask God for your healing so that you can live your life to the full potential, with purpose and meaning. You may not need healing to re-produce a physical child, but rather to give birth to a business, a ministry, a book or a maybe a new product. Whatever it may be, you can apply the principles and scriptures in this book until you receive your breakthrough. Are you ready to declare your healing? If so, allow these 77 verses to bring healing to your life and at the same time to the land.

Purpose of this Book

I could share about the history of Abraham and who he was and why God used Abraham to be the first person to introduce healing to mankind, after all, there were many before his time that God could have used to demonstrate his healing powers. However, for purposes of this book that is not significant because God wanted this book to be a quick read. He was specific that this book should be short, practical and straight to the point.

Nevertheless, it is worth mentioning that Abraham was a man of great faith and is often referred to as the Father of Faith. Abraham walked by faith and not by what he was seeing. He didn't allow his current circumstances to define his destiny. In fact, most times he did not know where he was going or what the outcome of a situation was going to be. He trusted the process and took one step at a time until he saw the promises he was believing for.

Healing is a process and can sometimes feel like an un-ending journey. Sometimes it is a quick immediate process and other times it's a long process. It all depends on God. For example, at one of my doctor's visit, it was discovered that I had a hernia and needed to have surgery to repair it. I didn't want to have surgery, so after leaving the doctor's office I immediately touched my stomach and prayed that I was healed and would not need the surgery. When I went back to the doctor's office for a follow-up appointment, the test results showed that I did not need surgery and that my hernia was completely healed.

On the other hand, some healing can be a longer process. After losing twin boys at 5 months' gestation and then a miscarriage, it was determined by the doctors (notice I said the doctors) that I had an incompetent cervix which is basically saying that my cervix dilates before its time. Long story short, I had to be on complete bedrest to have children. This bedrest was after God had promised me that I would be the mother of three children during my time of mourning after losing the twin boys.

Most times when God gives you a promise it's quite funny that He never really tells you the process. This bedrest became one of the best times I've had in my life because I got to know God for real. While I knew that I was healed at the beginning of the pregnancy, I still needed to go through the process. I still visited my doctor and did the things she said. I was on complete bedrest and I was obedient in making sure that while I was believing by faith in God, being steadfast and unmovable in Him, I still had to go through the process.

There were times during my routine checkup that the doctor kept saying that I was still dilating too quickly. Oh, forgot to mention that I had to get a cerclage (stitching of the cervix at 12 weeks' gestation). So even with all the medical interventions and the total bedrest there were moments and times when things still didn't look good. I was doing everything that was humanly possible to do, and leaving the rest up to God. God loves when we are totally dependent on Him. He loves being needed and He loves when at the end of the day, we can say had it not been for

God... I say all that to say that even though I knew I was healed, I still needed to go through the process as I kept the faith. I didn't waver. I got to a point that I knew that I was going to give birth to this child and that I was going to be the mother. He didn't tell me the process.

Our beautiful healthy daughter was born full term at a whopping 9lbs 11oz. This experience taught me how to not only give birth but the strategy to go through the process. My entire journey of birthing forth the children that were promised to me took almost 10 years in totality.

Your situation may be different, but it's just an example to demonstrate that as you are believing and praying to God for a healing and declaring the scriptures, you may also be required to take the necessary steps that are applicable for your situation. For example, if you need healing in your relationships, you can't just pray alone and leave it there. Well you can, but if you truly want to experience the full measure of healing, you must also seek ways to re-build that relationship or walk away from it if it's not healthy for you. Sometimes the healing process means closing a door to something and not wavering (going back and forth). You know your situation best, so apply the principle of faith and action as you go through the process.

I am not guaranteeing you that you will be healed by reading this book, but rather that it is your faith in God, His Word and the steps that you take to walk in and through His divine healing. The purpose of this book is to pull out the 77 scriptures in the bible that speak to healing that is a quick reference that you can use to decree and declare every day. I wish I had a book like this with quick scripture references when I was going through some difficult seasons in my life.

Use these 77 medicinal scriptures to declare healing in any area of your life, whether it's your physical health, financial health, spiritual health, relational health, etc. It doesn't matter what area. You can use this short book as your quick reference guide to declare the healing in your life, because the time is NOW! It's time to experience a healthy life and a healthy land. It's the right TIME!!! I will also be sharing excerpts and principles from my "Detox Your LiFE™" course from www.carolynganderson.com.

PART I – HEALTH

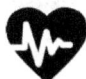

In the last few years it seems that there's been a pandemic (more than an epidemic) of people dying from various diseases especially cancer. These deaths range from the very young to the very old. It's as though it has become a virus (which it's not) that is traveling at great speed throughout the earth like a common cold. There are countries where cancer was pretty much non-existent and most people tend to die from natural causes when they reached a certain age.

Countries such as Jamaica, where when someone died, it was just from natural causes or maybe some form of heart disease or diabetes. Today almost one in every other death seems to be some form of cancer and it's not just affecting the senior citizens, but the young people are also dying from this dreadful disease. In the United States, childhood diseases are at an all-time high. I am convinced that there's something in the food, atmosphere, clothing and skin care products that is causing toxicity in our bodies that eventually lead to these diseases especially cancer.

Cancer attempted to show its ugly head in my life, when after a mammogram, I had to do an ultrasound of the breast because of an abnormality in the test results. I underwent a biopsy procedure where they ended up taking a sample of what they thought they saw and sent it off to the lab for testing. I recall laying there on the bed, looking up at the tiles in the ceiling and all I could see were that the tiles formed many points of interception that resembles a cross. I remember hearing a still small voice that said, "slow down Carolyn." I knew that this was God telling me to give Him the crosses in my life because I should not be carrying them on my own. I had so much going on and was so **busy** (the acronym for **being under satan's yoke**), and I needed to focus on my health because life is no good without a great health. Sometimes we can be so busy that we don't take time to care for ourselves. That is a trick of the enemy.

Everything I was doing at the time seemed necessary, such as being involved in the church, full time employment, running back and forth with the children, attending to my wifey duties, full time school and much more. How do you choose what to cut out when they all seem relevant? You might be going through a similar situation, where you don't know what to give up. Do what I did, I simply paused, assessed my life, and that's when I realized that I needed to detox and remove some toxins from my life (I will share more later about this process). You see this wasn't my first pause, however if you are not having a lot of self-reflection moments or taking time to evaluate your life often, the busyness of everyday life can take over.

While I had to go through the biopsy process, I was never worried at all, but it was indeed a wakeup call. Several years prior I wrote a verbal decree that stated that myself, my family and the generation after I are disease free and debt free. I gave no permission to anything to invade my body. You can do the same. If some form of disease be in mental, physical or spiritual have invaded your body, you can serve it notice and fire it! The principles and the stories I am sharing can be applied immediately. Each story or example I share is medicine, it is like a ground-breaking cure and treatment that starts now! The Bible says that we overcome by our testimonies and what God does for one, He can do it for the other. We have not even started decreeing the 77 scriptures, but already you should be feeling empowered and inspired that you can experience healing NOW.

Christ already paid the price and by His stripes you are healed. If you are a child of God, a believer and you have accepted Jesus Christ as your personal Lord and Savior, then it is illegal for any disease to be in your body. I strongly believe that some diseases are spirits because Jesus spent a lot of time casting out evil spirits and administering healing to those who needed it and two spirits cannot dwell in the same body. It must be one or the other. I am not saying that if someone has a disease or an illness that it's an evil spirit. What I am saying is that make a decree and declaration over your life that you are healed.

If you want healing and you want it bad enough and you're willing to get it, by all means necessary, then you must become radical, a warrior and fight if you are a child of God. You have the weapon to fight, which is the Word of God. You can declare that by His Stripes you are healed in Jesus Name. It doesn't matter what the illness or dis-ease may be. It can be terminal or it can be something that has an existing cure. The Bible says that all, not just some, but all diseases can be healed according to (Psalm 103:3 NIV…heals all your diseases). If you have a terminal disease, it's only (term-inal) by man's standards, which means that it's a term and it has an expiration date. Like life insurance policies there are term life and there's whole life policies, and with term life it has an expiration date but not with whole life. You can experience wholeness in Christ Jesus. Believe the word of God, He can heal any disease, any illness, any sickness, because He is the God that heals. If you have not accepted Jesus Christ as your personal Lord and Savior, you can do that now, so that you can have access to all His benefits, one of them being healed.

Moments of Reflection...................

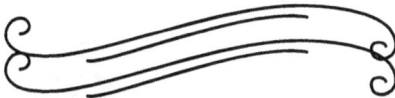

I want you to pause and take a moment and reflect on your life. Write a new decree about your health. Write your declaration and denounce any disease that you may have.

_____

_____

_____

_____

_____

PART II - FINANCE

$

One of the unhealthiest areas of life can be found in your finances. With today's economic turmoil, uncertainties, people's income falling below the poverty level, there is a desperate need for healing in the areas of finance. Money is needed for pretty much everything. Money is needed for food, shelter and clothing. The worlds' economic system is built around finances and earth's currency is fueled by money. What I mean by that is everything comes with a price, whether it's buying food, caring for your health, having money to pay bills, tithing, maintaining your relationships or saving for a rainy day per se. Everything comes with a price and someone is financing it one way or another.

According to Ecclesiastes 10:19 NIV it states, *"A feast is made for laughter, wine makes life merry, and money is the answer for everything"* however, 1 Timothy 6:10 states *"For the love of money is a root of all kinds of evil. Some people, eager for money, have wandered from the faith and pierced themselves with many griefs."* Loving money more than you love God and making it like a god is where it becomes evil. When you put anything before God it is evil. Some people worship and serve their money. It means everything to them and when they lose it, they pretty much lose their life.

Yet others have dealt with their finances in the best way possible, but it also appears that there's still a lack. Some monetary problems could have transferred down generation to generation. If you are not sure whether your problem is generational or not, I would suggest that you take this time and pray and ask God to heal you from any generational curse that may have transferred from previous generations that is affecting your finance. Just like in any area of life, you can receive healing in your finance.

My husband and I have witnessed God's healing virtue in our finances. During the first years of our marriage, we maintained a healthy financial record of where the money was going. I managed the day to day operations of our accounts and he was responsible for the long-term investments. We worked well together and at the end of each year, after paying our property taxes and all bills we always ended up with money in our savings account.

In addition to having a savings account, we were also very strict tithers and always gave a 10th of our earnings to the church. We took vacations to wherever we wanted to go, had great jobs and lived a pretty stabled life with the option to purchase anything we wanted because we also had great credit scores. As time went on and we started accumulating more, having children and economic changes, things started going downhill.

During the housing market downfall in 2008, we purchased what some would call a dream home. I didn't realize that there was a recession going on because I don't participate in the world's system but rather the kingdom. Nevertheless, we moved into our dream home and placed the other home on the market for sale. Unfortunately, we ended up with two mortgages for two years, caring for two little ones and things became difficult. It got harder and harder to stay on top of things and we had to rely on our credit cards to pay some of our bills.

Consequently, this financial strain started affecting our marriage and we started having arguments about finances. Prior to this downfall, we never argued about money and always had more than enough. We started living pay-check to pay-check and even though I had switched jobs and was now making six figures plus my husband's income we were still having problems and living paycheck to paycheck. It became so bad that we pretty much became bankrupt and needed healing in our finances. The financial problems were so severe and it was not only affecting our relationship between each other but also my physical health. I was desperate for a change and something had to be done.

If you recall when I needed physical healing in my body, I not only believed God for a healing, but also took some necessary steps in the process. The same is true for healing in finances. First I prayed and asked God for healing in our finances. I then wrote a decree and declaration that our finances are healed and that we are debt free. I learned that when you owe anyone (banks, people, credit card companies) money, that you are a slave (Proverbs 22:7 NIV). I didn't want to be a slave, so we put together a debt free plan that would get us out of debt and live a life of abundance in our finances.

We became very intentional about the finances and implemented a debt free and wealth creation strategy. We created a strict budget and every dime needed to be accounted for. We had messed up big time and allowed our finances to get out of control and we needed God to forgive us as we put forth a financial plan that would get us out of debt and allowed us to live a life of freedom.

God is so merciful and gracious and loves to see us experience his love through being healed. The Heavenly Father desires that you are healed in your finances and that you have more than enough. He is the God of more than enough. It is not His will that you would be living paycheck to paycheck, never having enough and always limited by resources. You should be able to live a fruitful life and have enough for everything. You should be the lender and not the borrower. You are the one that people should be coming to when they want to borrow and not the other way around. You should be able to live life more abundantly and to live it fully every day. Are you ready to be set free from the system of financial slavery?

Moments of Reflection..................

Pause and take a moment to reflect: Write down the areas of your finances that needs healing..........Secondly, write your declaration of what you want your financial health to look like.

_____

_____

_____

_____

_____

_____

_____

_____

_____

PART III - FAITH

Just as one may need healing in his or her health or finance, sometimes their needs to be healing in the areas of faith. This area is rather tricky because sometimes one isn't aware that he or she is hurting in their faith. The main reason for this is because the pains, hurts and scars associated with faith cannot be seen with the naked eye. Faith is a spiritual matter and cannot be seen, so unlike needing physical healing or financial healing which can be seen, when it comes to your faith it cannot be seen with the naked eye.

Faith is also multifaceted, because it includes matters of the heart, the mind, the spirit and the soul. It embodies elements of hopelessness, the belief system, values, inherited traits and an entire gamete of emotions. Typically, the awareness of hurting in your faith tends to be revealed when there's what I call a (pause) moment.

Pause Button

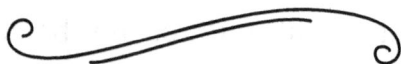

A pause moment is when life hits the pause button and you're forced to stop. Something happens that makes you stop and evaluate your life and truly get in touch with your feelings. Pausing tends to be easier for females than it is for males, perhaps because most women are more emotional than men and women like to have an answer for life's situations. It's probably the latter (lol). A woman will evaluate her life to understand the root of the pain, more so than men, but not all.

Without this pause moment life just keeps going and going and going until one day when something forces a STOP! A PAUSE! If you don't (pause) on you own, if you don't deal with the matter, then God will pause you and you don't want that. His pauses can be very abrupt. God is such a gentleman that He doesn't speak in the noise. He waits until you're done with your everyday hustle and bustle and able to listen and hear Him without interruption. According to Bishop T.D. Jakes, "You can't hear in the noise and if "you can't hear, you can't heal." Sometimes you will need to take a step back and have moments of reflection, if your faith has been shaken.

I know the pause moment very well. I've had several pause moments. From being on bedrest, to losing a job, homelessness, marital problems to being hospitalized waiting to give birth to a child, and so much more. Some of these pause moments are longer than others. Most times while in the pause moments they are never pleasant and you never really see the benefit until you're out of them. Most recently, I experienced a very traumatic pause moment or more like a

PAUSE SEASON. It was moments on top of moments and they were coming from everywhere nonstop. From my college advisor for my doctoral program turning against me and the university dismissing me, to investing in expensive coaching programs and having nothing to show for it, not even a certificate, to people who I have helped in the past suddenly are nowhere to be found when I needed help. I was hurting deeply, so deeply that there were times that I felt like I was slowly dying. There were times when I wanted to simply give up. I felt like I was in a lifetime movie that is a sequel and it's not ending. I didn't see the light in this pause moment (season). I was in utter shock and dis-belief that so many things were happening to me at the same time and I didn't understand why. The pain ran so deep that I felt like my soul was wounded.

Soul Wounds

Wounded soul! What's that? I didn't realize that a soul could be wounded and need healing. You have a wounded soul when you're struggling to find words to express how you feel. The pain is indescribable. It's a state of hopelessness. I was heartbroken repeatedly until the pain ran so deep that it caused the soul to be scarred and needed to be repaired. I believe that there are lots of people out there that aren't even aware that their soul need healing. I didn't know! I didn't even know that there was such a thing. It wasn't until I was crying out to God asking Him what's going on with me, why do I feel this way and just like the gentle Father that He, he whispered "your soul is hurting." I understood being heart broken and I understood emotional hurt. I understood physical hurt and relational hurt, but soul hurting was a new concept for me.

Soul hurting is the deepest form of hurt. It runs really deep and it's normally developed over time. It can be years. For some people, it goes back to childhood. This hurt is more than just your faith being shaken, or having a few disappointments. This is when your life has been so shattered that you feel numb. It's a state of hopelessness and deep despair. It's when life becomes neutral and you're simply existing. For me, this was rather deep, because I had lost passion for life, which is not normal for me. I'm very passionate and I love (hard), meaning that when I love or like you, I give you my all. I don't know how to give just a little or even 90%, I wish I did, but it's just not in my DNA. So, this deep hurting needed to be healed, because it was affecting the very core of who I was created to be. If you are feeling anything close to what I am expressing, it is possible that you need healing in your soul and your faith has been shaken. If you are experiencing anxiety, frustration, anger and at times difficulty concentrating, then chances are your soul is wounded. With so many wounded souls, it leads to a wounded nation.

The Soul of a Nation

This is the problem that the world is experiencing NOW, especially in the United States of America. The soul of the nation is wounded. The souls of the people that make up the nation are wounded. There's anxiety, anger, frustration, death, violence and deep soul pains. It runs deep and slapping a band-aid on the problem will not heal the deep wounds. It just covers them temporarily. Just like when the body experiences a deep wound, you may put a band-aid over it to prevent re-injury or from it being exposed, but deep down the wound is still there and it's not healed. Exposure brings closure!

In the military, I was taught that exposing some injuries or allowing it to breathe for a period, speeds up the healing process. If a wound is not dealt with properly and not cared for in the right way, it may appear that all is well, but deep down it's not healed.

This is what's happening in our world today. It appears that multiple wounds, deep soul wounds are being covered up with Band-Aids and that's not going to solve the problems. We must find the root of the problem, dig it up, deal with it, expose it and start the healing process of re-pairing, re-planting and re-building.

One of the first steps to deal with the problem is through prayer and talking about it. According to 2 Chronicles 7:14 NIV is says *"if my people, who are called by my name, will humble themselves and pray and seek my face and turn from their wicked ways, then I will hear from heaven, and I will forgive their sin and will heal their land."*

The Land is desperately in need of healing and it requires praying, seeking God and turning from our wicked ways. The unhealthy soul of the nation is causing a ripple effect. A nation, a family, an organization are all made up of people and when individuals are hurting, it affects marriages, families, communities and then become widespread to affect nations and society at large. Therefore, your healing is so necessary because transformation starts with just one person at a time. Your healing is the beginning of the change that's needed in the world today.

You may have lost faith in yourself, in God, in your leaders and you're probably shaken right now, but know that all wounds can be healed. The areas of pain must be dealt with to its fullness so that the healing process can begin to take place. Your faith can be restored and you can live again. You can believe again; you can hope again. You can live a healthy, prosperous and great life. You can have that Faith to believe the impossible. Don't settle for the status quo and a mediocre life. You can remove the limitations. Your dreams can live, your visions can become a reality, your faith can be restored, believe it and you can receive it. You are royalty, you are a chosen generation, you can rise above the lack of hope and lack of faith if you just believe. Be healed!

Moments of Reflection..................

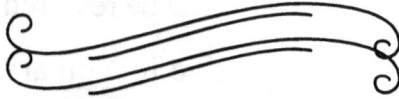

Pause and take a moment to reflect on your Faith. Has it been shaken in anyway? Thereafter take a moment and complete the exercise below..........

I have found that one of the places that our faith becomes wounded is in our belief system. Our thoughts become what we believe and what we believe is portrayed through our actions. Our thoughts can be toxic without us knowing it and it's developed over time through the belief system. Do you have empowering or dis-empowering beliefs? Beliefs are a feeling of certainty around what a thing means.

Like values, your beliefs motivate you and impact your life. You collect your beliefs, usually subconsciously, from your friends, family and society, and from your experiences. It is usually easier to radically change a belief than it is to radically change a value, because beliefs come from interpreting an event at a specific point in time.

EXAMPLE: Changing Values versus Changing Beliefs

It is harder to go from valuing 'health' to valuing 'illness,' and easier to go from believing that you are 'unfit' to believing that you are 'healthy.'

Beliefs can be totally empowering or totally disempowering (see example below). Most people are carrying around many disempowering beliefs that bring them down every day and they don't even know it...Therefore, are part of the healing process, it is very possible that you can change your life and be healed, but changing your belief system.

How many disempowering and empowering beliefs are you carrying around with you? Let's look at your beliefs and make sure that they all serve, support, and nurture you.

Examples

Disempowering Belief

I will never get ahead

I always mess things up

Empowering Belief

I always learn something when I try something new

I am smart and intelligent

In this healing process, let's focus on what's important to you. You can ONLY do so successful if you remove thoughts and mindsets that are not good for you. This way you will be able to have room for positive thinking.

"Whether you think you can or whether you think you can't, you are right." Henry Ford

Now I want you to do the below exercise by writing down the words below and completing the sentences.

Explore some of your beliefs by completing the following sentences.

Note: 'They' could represent your family, work colleagues or friends. 'She/He' could represent someone who is important to you like you mother/father, daughter/son, sister/brother, friend, etc.

My beliefs:

I always...

I never...

They are...

I can't...

We are...

I must...

I must...

My work is...

My time is...

My team is...

There are times when I...

Life is all about...

I love...

Success is...

Teamwork is...

Life is...

Family is...

Love is...

She can...

She is...

My parents are...

He could...

He is...

I am...

They are...

I can...

I can...

I can...

Empowering or Disempowering?

Take a few minutes to review your responses to each of the previous phrases. Write a 'D' next to each belief that is disempowering and an 'E' next to each belief that is empowering.

What does the previous exercise tell you about your beliefs?

_____

_____

_____

_____

_____

_____

_____

_____

What empowering beliefs do you have?

_____

_____

_____

_____

_____

_____

_____

_____

What can you replace your dis-empowering beliefs with?

_____

_____

_____

_____

_____

_____

_____

_____

PART IV – RELATIONSHIPS

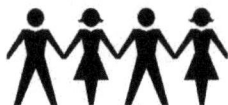

Broken relationships - this is one of the most overlooked area in life that requires healing. One of the reasons why relational brokenness is not so apparent is because it's typical healing in the emotions which cannot be seen. The scars that are in the heart from emotional or verbal abuse cannot be seen with the naked eye, because they are internal. Sometimes one may not even be aware that there's trauma until years later when what was buried surfaces. Oftentimes most interpersonal relationship problems are derivatives from other problems from previous relationships. What tends to happen is this pattern of not dealing with problems becomes a learned behavior and the individual isn't even aware there's a problem because he or she operates in survival mode.

Survival mode is when an individual just functions and acts as if nothing is really bothering him or her. They shut down the pain internally, so that they don't feel. That individual can be very functional at their occupation, but at home or with interpersonal relationships, he or she is failing miserably. I see this a lot in marriages especially with the spouse that is more reserved.

I've experienced this in my own marriage, where it was as though my husband was two different people. At work and at church, he's a high energetic individual, but he gets home and shuts down. This went on for years and I thought nothing of it, because I just assumed it was just personality differences. It wasn't until I started taking some mini-pause moments (remember the pause moments), and that's when I started saying something isn't right. I am married, yet I felt alone. To make a long story short, what we eventually discovered what that there was a childhood trauma issue, that was never dealt with and had caused my husband to become emotionally disconnected deep down and that required healing. This disconnection led me to become hurt so deep because I had spent so much time and energy seeking a solution for my husband and the pain of feeling like the marriage for him was just a formality was shattering and I was wounded.

When my husband finally accepted that there was a problem, that's when his healing started and then we went through the process to re-building. It wasn't easy and it did take a while to recover. There were lots of arguments, name calling, defenses and offenses. It wasn't pretty.

Today, however, I am grateful for the experiences and would not trade them for anything. My husband has matured into such a phenomenal visionary, leader, father, husband and friend. He's now free and healed to the point of energetically sharing his story. His profound book (The Fatherless Father) touches on some of the healing that he experienced and the blessings that comes with a healed heart. The exposure of the problems brought closure. A relationship whether mother and child, spouses, best friends, etc., must be tested and only the strong ones will survive.

Every relationship will come to a point where there's a conflict, where there's a choice to be made. It comes to a point where the authenticity and strength of the relationship undergoes a test. Some tests are long and some are short. This is when you truly get to see others for who they are and when they show who you they are. Believe it when it's shown. If the relationship is valuable and worth continuing, then both parties must do all that's necessary to save that relationship.

The process may be a little bumpy but healing in relationships takes time. This is one of the areas of life that you cannot rush. If you rush the process, it may be detrimental. The first step to healing in any relationship is forgiveness and forgiveness itself is also a process. Please note that forgiveness does not mean that you forget the situation and that you're all in again. Forgiveness is for you, so that you don't harbor resentment, hate or anger. Harboring those things will keep you in the shadows of the past and you don't want that because it's your time to be FREE!

There are some relationships that forgiveness means that you move on. These are the relationships that are toxic and not healthy for you and not going anywhere. You know best what is right for you and God has given you the freedom to make choices – so choose well. According to Gladwell (2008), in his book Outliers, he said that "the people we surround ourselves with have a profound effect on who we are" (p.11), so therefore it's imperative that you are surrounded by the right people that's suitable for your life.

.

Your healing and your new life starts today!

Moments of Reflection...................

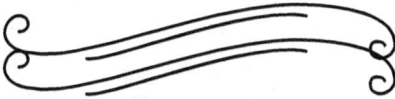

Pause and take a moment to reflect: Write down any broken relationships that still needs healing or forgiveness..........

_____

_____

_____

_____

_____

Summary

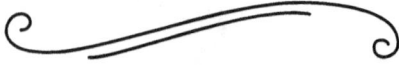

As you prepare to decree and declare these 77 scriptures over your life, there's a very important step that is the pre-requisite before your declarations. To receive these benefits, you must first be a son or daughter of the Highest God. One of the benefits of being a child of God is that you get complete access to His healing, plus many more benefits. In a moment, you will have the opportunity to say a simple prayer that will give you access Father through His Son Jesus Christ.

Years ago, my father had prostate cancer and he underwent surgery to remove the cancer. For about two years everything was fine and it appeared that my dad was cured or in remission as some call in. Tragically the cancer came back or came back from hiding and this time it was more potent and powerful than the first time. His doctors pretty much said that there was nothing else they can do for him. He was just told to get regular checkups and hope that something changed. Thus, his disease became a death sentence waiting and hoping for a healing miracle.

My husband and I are both Pastors and one Sunday after I ministered and gave an open invitation for an altar call, to my surprise my dad came to the altar. Growing up, I never saw my dad attend church, but he always made sure that we went to church. The only time I saw him at a church service was at a funeral and I don't recall him being inside the church. He mostly hung outside. We grew up in Jamaica and it was mostly over 80 degrees so being outside was never a problem for him or anyone that wanted to be outside.

This Sunday something happened. I believed my dad was the last person that I prayed for. Prior to praying for him, I asked my dad if he was saved. I asked him if he had ever received Jesus Christ as his personal Lord and Savior. He had not, so then I asked him if he would like to be saved? Without hesitation, he said yes. After my father accepted Jesus Christ as his savior, I did something I have never done before. I looked directly at my father and said, "it is illegal for two spirits to dwell in the same body, therefore I command the spirit of cancer to leave his body now, because the Holy Spirit now lives there." The following day was one of my dad's regular checkups for the cancer levels in his body.

Long story short, to their amazing surprise there was no cancer. To this day, my dad is healed from cancer and enjoying his life playing golf and traveling. My point is when the earthly doctors have reached a point when they can do nothing else for you and if you're a child of God, that's when you turn to the Heavenly Doctor who can do the impossible.

There's nothing too hard for God and when you have accepted His Son it gives you direct access to receive all the benefits from him. It's no different from the places of employment how they each come with standard benefits such as health insurance. So, it is when you are in Christ Jesus, there are standard benefits that comes with being a part of the kingdom and one of those is healing. I should also point out that my dad also took the necessary steps thereafter and started to live a healthier life by eating the proper nutrition and exercising regularly. Being healed doesn't mean that you will not have to maintain a healthy lifestyle, because you will. You must take care of the temple, the finances, the relationships, and the mind that God has given you. Faith and works always work together. So, you must not only believe but you must also take action steps to a live a life of wholeness. Are you ready to live life fully every day?

Confession

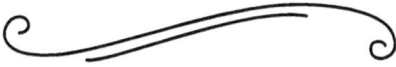

It's a simple process that takes less than 5 minutes. It's a three-step process as easy as ABC!

1. Accept Jesus Christ as your Lord and Savior
2. Believe in your heart that He died for you and that He is the risen savior that will return
3. Confess your sins and ask him to forgive you and forgive others as well

Congratulations! If you have just accepted Jesus Christ as your personal Lord & Savior, you can now fully participate in the blessings that are in store for you.

Date of Salvation: _____

77 Scriptures for Healing

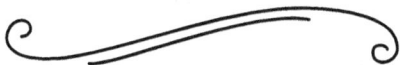

Now it's time to decree and declare the word of God in any area of your life. According to Job 22:28, it states that you shall decree a thing and it shall be established in your life. Therefore, decree these scriptures over your life. Make them very personal to your situation. For example, you can state that: *I decree and declare that I am healed according to Genesis 20:17 where Abraham prayed to you and you healed Abimelech and his family and since you are the same God then, today and forevermore, I am praying for a healing and I believe that I am healed*. You can personalize the scriptures as you see fit and receive your healing.

Let your healing begin...

#1 - Genesis 20:17 AMP

So, Abraham prayed to God, and God healed Abimelech and his wife and his female slaves, and they bore children...

(Which means that the ability to not produce or to not reproduce requires healing) Abimelech's reproductive seed was re-routed or shut off and so were the females around him, and when Abraham prayed and asked God for healing God healed him and his family. This is the first place that healing is mentioned in the bible. The year 2017 initiates your healing.

#2 - Exodus 15:26 AMP

...If you will diligently hearken to the voice of the Lord your God and will do what is right in His sight, and will listen to and obey His commandments and keep all His statutes, I will put none of the diseases upon you which I brought upon the Egyptians, for I am the Lord Who heals you.

#3 - Exodus 23:25-26 MSG

But you---you serve your God and he'll bless your food and your water. I'll get rid of the sickness among you; there won't be any miscarriages nor barren women in your land. I'll make sure you live full and complete lives.

#4 - Exodus 23:25 AMP

You shall serve the Lord your God; He shall bless your bread and water, and I will take sickness from your midst.

#5 - Numbers 12:13 AMP

And Moses cried to the Lord, saying, Heal her now, O God, I beseech You!

Cry out to the Lord if you need a healing NOW! He's listening and waiting to hear your prayers and to heal you.

#6 - Deuteronomy 32:39 AMP

See now that I, I am He, and there is no god beside Me; I kill and I make alive, I wound and I heal, and there is none who can deliver out of My hand.

#7 - 2 Kings 20:5 AMP

...Thus says the Lord, the God of David your forefather: I have heard your prayer, I have seen your tears; behold, I will heal you...

#8 - 2 Chronicles 7:14 AMP

If My people, who are called by My name, shall humble themselves, pray, seek, crave, and require of necessity My face and turn from their wicked ways, then will I hear from heaven, forgive their sin, and heal their land.

#9 - 2 Chronicles 30:20 AMP

And the Lord hearkened to Hezekiah and healed the people.

#10 - Job 5:18 AMP

For He wounds, but He binds up; He smites, but His hands heal.

#11 - Psalm 6:2 AMP

Have mercy on me and be gracious to me, O Lord, for I am weak (faint and withered away); O Lord, heal me, for my bones are troubled.

#12 - Psalm 30:2 AMP

O Lord my God, I cried to You and You have healed me.

Make this healing word very personal to your situation. At the end of the declaration you can add, ...you have healed me in my finances, marriage, cancer, etc., (make it personal to your situation). I decree and declare that I cried out to you and you have healed me from (_____) or healed my marriage, finance, emotions, etc.

#13 - Psalm 41:4 AMP

I said, Lord, be merciful and gracious to me; heal my inner self, for I have sinned against You.

#14 - Psalm 103:3 AMP

Who forgives every one of all your iniquities, who heals each one of all your diseases,

Decree and declare that according to Psalm 103:3, all your diseases are healed

#15 - Psalm 107:20 AMP

He sends forth His word and heals them and rescues them from the pit and destruction.

#16 - Psalm 119:37 AMP

...Restore me to vigorous life and health in Your ways.

Decree and declare that you are restored to a good life and that you are healthy according to Psalm 119:37

#17 - Psalm 147:3 AMP

He heals the brokenhearted and binds up their wounds curing their pains and their sorrows.

Decree and declare that you are healed from a broken heart and that you have bind up your wounds according to Psalm 147:3

#18 - Proverbs 12:18 AMP

There are those who speak rashly, like the piercing of a sword, but the tongue of the wise brings healing.

#19 - Proverbs 13:17 AMP

A wicked messenger falls into evil, but a faithful ambassador brings healing.

#20 - Proverbs 15:30 NIV

Light in a messenger's eyes brings joy to the heart, and good news gives health to the bones.

Decree and declare that today you will have joy in your heart and that you will receive good news and healing in your body according to Proverbs 15:30

#21 - Ecclesiastes 3:3 NIV

a time to kill and a time to heal, a time to tear down and a time to build, ...

Decree and declare that NOW is your time to be healed according to Ecclesiastes 3:3

#22 - Isaiah 38:16 NIV

…You restored me to health and let me live.

Decree and declare that God has restored to you good health and allows you to live according to Isaiah 38:16

#23 - Isaiah 53:5 NIV

But he was pierced for our transgressions, he was crushed for our iniquities; the punishment that brought us peace was on him, and by his wounds we are healed.

Decree and declare that Jesus Christ already paid the price and that by His stripes you are healed.

#24 - Isaiah 57:18-19 NIV

I have seen their ways, but I will heal them; I will guide them and restore comfort …," says the Lord. "And I will heal them."

#25 - Isaiah 58:8 NIV

Then your light will break forth like the dawn, and your healing will quickly appear; then your righteousness will go before you, and the glory of the Lord will be your rear guard.

Decree and declare that your healing comes quickly and will not be delayed according to Isaiah 58:8

#26 - Jeremiah 17:14 NIV

Heal me, Lord, and I will be healed; save me and I will be saved, for you are the one I praise.

Decree and declare that you are healed and that God has saved you according to Jeremiah 17:14

#27 - Jeremiah 30:17 NIV

But I will restore you to health and heal your wounds,' declares the Lord, 'because you are called an outcast, Zion for whom no one cares.'

The Lord loves you. It doesn't matter what you have done or even what you have been through, the Lord loves you. He shed his blood so that you don't have to. You may be considered an outcast, different, abused, abandoned, talked about, rejected, hopeless, feeling like you deserve what you are going through, but the Lord has declared that He will re-store you to health and heal the inner and outer WOUNDS. Jesus Christ already paid the price so that you can be HEALED! Receive His GIFT! Decree and Declare that you are healed.

#28 - Jeremiah 33:6 NIV

"Nevertheless, I will bring health and healing to it; I will heal my people and will let them enjoy abundant peace and security.

What the Lord is saying is that it doesn't matter that you have wronged him or others. If you seek forgiveness and repent, He will heal you. I decree and declare that I am healed and that I live an abundant and healed life with added peace and security.

#29 - Hosea 14:4 NIV

"I will heal their waywardness and love them freely, for my anger has turned away from them.

Say out Loud: I decree and declare that God is not angry with you and that you are healed

#30 - Matthew 4:23 NIV

Jesus went throughout Galilee, teaching in their synagogues, proclaiming the good news of the kingdom, and healing every disease and sickness among the people.

He is the same Jesus then, today and forevermore. If He healed the people in Galilee, he will heal you today. I decree and declare that I am healed for every disease and sickness whether in my health, finance, faith or relationships according to Matthew 4:23

#31 - Matthew 4:24 NIV

News about him spread all over Syria, and people brought to him all who were ill with various diseases, those suffering severe pain, the demon-possessed, those having seizures, and the paralyzed; and he healed them.

#32 - Matthew 6:22 NIV

"The eye is the lamp of the body. If your eyes are healthy, your whole body will be full of light.

See your healing through the eyes of the Father. He cares for you and loves you very much and I pray that God give you the eyes to see how much He desires healing in every area of your life.

#33 - Matthew 8:8, 8:13 NIV

The centurion replied, "Lord, I do not deserve to have you come under my roof. But just say the word, and my servant will be healed. Then Jesus said to the centurion, "Go! Let it be done just as you believed it would." And his servant was healed at that moment.

You may feel like you're not worthy for Jesus to be in your spiritual home or that you don't deserve to be saved or to be loved, but The Lord is saying I love you. These scriptures are MEDICINE that God has sent to you, so receive His healing.

#34 - Matthew 8:16-17 NIV

When evening came, many who were demon-possessed were brought to him, and he drove out the spirits with a word and healed all the sick. [17] This was to fulfill what was spoken through the prophet Isaiah: "He took up our infirmities and bore our diseases."

At the name of Jesus Christ, even the demons must flee. No matter what troubles have plague your home or what bloodline curse may have surrounded you, just declare that you are healed and you shall be healed.

#35 - Matthew 9:22 NIV

Jesus turned and saw her. "Take heart, daughter," he said, "your faith has healed you." And the woman was healed at that moment.

INSTANT HEALING - are you looking for an instant Healing? Do you need a miracle in your life right now? Just like Jesus did for this woman, He can do the same for you whether you're a man or woman. Activate your faith, trust and believe in Him and receive your healing.

#36 - Matthew 9:35 NIV

Jesus went through all the towns and villages, teaching in their synagogues, proclaiming the good news of the kingdom and healing every disease and sickness.

Don't allow what Jesus did for you to be in vain. He went through the process of dying for you and I so that through his death we may have life. He already redeemed you from illnesses and diseases. It doesn't matter what the illness it, He said every disease is healed. When man does not have a cure, Jesus said "you are healed."

#37 - Matthew 10:1 NIV

Jesus called his twelve disciples to him and gave them authority to drive out impure spirits and to heal every disease and sickness.

If you are in Christ Jesus, you are one of his disciples. Therefore, lay hands on your own body and decree and declare your healing.

#38 - Matthew 10:8 NIV

Heal the sick, raise the dead, cleanse those who have leprosy, drive out demons. Freely you have received; freely give.

Once you have received your healing, it's now time to help someone else.

#39 - Matthew 12:15 NIV

…. A large crowd followed him, and he healed all who were ill.

If you want to be healed, follow Jesus and be a part of His crowd.

#40 - Matthew 12:22 NIV

Then they brought him a demon-possessed man who was blind and mute, and Jesus healed him, so that he could both talk and see.

The blind can see and the deaf can hear and the dumb can speak. It doesn't matter what the disease is or the situation may look like. Jesus Christ can heal them all.

Are you spiritually blind? Decree and declare that you are no longer blind, dumb, deaf or hard of hearing, because now you can talk, see, hear, and feel according to Matthew 12:22

#41- Matthew 14:14 NIV

When Jesus landed, and saw a large crowd, he had compassion on them and healed their sick.

Jesus has compassion for you so receive your healing.

#42 - Matthew 14:36 NIV

….and all who touched it were healed.

Touch Jesus and you shall be healed

#43 - Matthew 15:28 NIV

Then Jesus said to her, "Woman, you have great faith! Your request is granted." And her daughter was healed at that moment.

You can pray for others to be healed as well as others can pray for you to be healed. You can also ask others to pray with you for your healing. I touch and agree that the healing you need shall come to you in Jesus Name.

#44 - Matthew 15:30 NIV

"Great crowds came to him, bringing the lame, the blind, the crippled, the mute and many others, and laid them at his feet; and he healed them."

It doesn't matter what area of your life that you need healing in. Your finances may be crippled, your health may be mute, your relationships may be lame, and your faith may be shattered, Jesus can heal it all. You must decree it, believe it, and you shall receive it.

#45 - Matthew 17:18 NIV

"Jesus rebuked the demon, and it came out of the boy, and he was healed at that moment."

If you are in Christ Jesus and the Holy Spirit lives and dwells within you and you have another spirit (such as cancer or HIV or any illnesses) that is invading your body, that spirit is operating on illegal terms, because two (2) spirits cannot dwell within the same body, it must be one or the other. Therefore, use the HEALING WORDS of God to bind and rebuke anything within your life that does not line up with the will of God.

#46 - Matthew 19:2 NIV

Large crowds followed him, and he healed them there.

Decree and declare that you are a follower of Jesus Christ therefore you are healed according to Matthew 19:2

#47 - Matthew 21:14 NIV

The blind and the lame came to him at the temple, and he healed them.

If you are physically or spiritually blind, meaning you're not able to see out of your physical eyes or you're not able to see from your mind because your problems have overtaken you, use this scripture to declare your healing.

#48 - Mark 1:34 NIV

...Jesus healed many who had various diseases.

Jesus can heal any dis-ease that you have. It may not be a physical disease, perhaps it's an emotional issue you are facing. Perhaps you are being bombarded with life's many problems and it's too much to bear. Jesus can cleanse you from all dis-ease.

#49 - Mark 3:10 NIV

For he had healed many, so that those with diseases were pushing forward to touch him.

How much do you want to be healed? If you want it bad enough, then PUSH through your current circumstances. Look beyond what people may be saying and trust and believe God. When I was pregnant with my son AJ, I had an episode where I was hemorrhaging and had to seek emergency care. The doctor didn't even bother to look at me. He saw the blood, and said that there's no viable life in my womb. I knew otherwise and even though I couldn't feel or see my son, I pushed beyond what the doctors were saying and trust and believe that I was healed. Today he's almost 7 years old. Don't believe the VOICES that are negative. Don't believe the negative report, trust GOD!

#50 - Mark 10:52 NIV

"Go," said Jesus, "your faith has healed you." Immediately he received his sight and followed Jesus along the road.

Your faith can move mountains, even if you are a new babe in Christ. All you need is faith to believe. I decree and declare that my faith in God has caused me to be healed.

#51 - Luke 4:40 NIV

At sunset, the people brought to Jesus all who had various kinds of sickness, and laying his hands on each one, he healed them.

Allow Jesus to touch you with His healing hands. Cry out to the Lord and let Him know that you need HIM!

#52 - Luke 5:15 NIV

Yet the news about him spread all the more, so that crowds of people came to hear him and to be healed of their sicknesses.

Will you listen to the Fox News, CNN, ABC or the Good NEWS? The Good News came and died and rose and He's sitting at the right hand of the father, making daily intercessions for you and I. I can't wait for you to spread the good news of your healing.

#53 - Luke 6:18 NIV

"who had come to hear him and to be healed of their diseases."

Decree and declare that you have come as far as you know and that you are healed from every illness in Jesus Name according to Luke 6:18

#54 - Luke 6:19 NIV

"and the people all tried to touch him, because power was coming from him and healing them all."

#55 - Luke 7:3 NIV

The centurion heard of Jesus and sent some elders of the Jews to him, asking him to come and heal his servant.

You don't have to send for Jesus anymore because He is right there wherever you are.

#56 - Luke 8:47-48 NIV

"Then the woman, seeing that she could not go unnoticed, came trembling and fell at his feet. In the presence of all the people, she told why she had touched him and how she had been instantly healed". Then he said to her, "Daughter, your faith has healed you. Go in peace."

#57 - Luke 8:50 NIV

Hearing this, Jesus said to Jairus, "Don't be afraid; just believe, and she will be healed."

Just believe and you shall be healed. Healing will not come to you if you do not believe. You have nothing to lose, so trust and believe that Jesus loves you and desires for you to be healed.

#58 - Luke 9:2 NIV

"and he sent them out to proclaim the kingdom of God and to heal the sick."

You can be healed

#59 - Luke 9:6 NIV

"So they set out and went from village to village, proclaiming the good news and healing people everywhere."

#60 - Luke 9:11 NIV

"but the crowds learned about it and followed him. He welcomed them and spoke to them about the kingdom of God, and healed those who needed healing."

How great is your need to be healed? Decree and declare that you are healed according to Luke 9:11. Surely 9/11 in the United States will always be a day to remember as one of the most devastating day in history. I believe that even today healing can still come to those that need healing and the land can be healed. We need healing.

#61 - Luke 9:42 NIV

Even while the boy was coming, the demon threw him to the ground in a convulsion. But Jesus rebuked the impure spirit, healed the boy and gave him back to his father.

You may feel as though you are knocked down to the ground. You may feel hopeless, helpless, broken, forgotten, abandoned, discouraged, afraid or fearful, but know that you can be healed from all disease or sickness.

#62 - Luke 10:9 NIV

Heal the sick who are there and tell them, 'The kingdom of God has come near to you.'

#63 - Luke 17:15 NIV

"One of them, when he saw he was healed, came back, praising God in a loud voice."

Be the one that praises God after your healing. Share your healing with someone else and let them know what God has done for you. I pray that you're the one! Be healed in Jesus Name.

#64 - Luke 18:42 NIV

Jesus said to him, "Receive your sight; your faith has healed you."

#65 - Luke 22:51 NIV

But Jesus answered, "No more of this!" And he touched the man's ear and healed him.

I pray that your hearing will be healed and that you can hear what God is saying to you beyond the noise. You may not be physically deaf, it could be a spiritual deafness, where you cannot hear what God is telling you to do. Are you walking daily in your divine purpose or are you deaf to the things of God. I decree and declare that I can hear clearly and I am healed according to Luke 22:51

#66 - John 4:47 NIV

When this man heard that Jesus had arrived in Galilee from Judea, he went to him and begged him to come and heal his son, who was close to death.

Do you feel like you're close to death? Do you know someone who may be close to death? According to this scripture, even if you are close to death, you can be healed. There's nothing impossible with God. Repent, Confess, Believe and be healed.

#67 - John 6:2 NIV

and a great crowd of people followed him because they saw the signs he had performed by healing the sick.

#68 - Acts 3:16 NIV

By faith in the name of Jesus, this man whom you see and know was made strong. It is Jesus' name and the faith that comes through him that has completely healed him, as you can all see.

In the name of Jesus, be healed!

#69 - Acts 4:22 NIV

For the man who was miraculously healed was over forty years old.

It doesn't matter your age, healing has no age restriction. Healing comes to the unborn, the young, middle aged or the old.

#70 - Acts 4:30 NIV

"Stretch out your hand to heal and perform signs and wonders through the name of your holy servant Jesus."

Through the name of Jesus, you can receive healing. You can lay your own hand on yourself, your bills and debts, your heart, your mind, body and declare your healing. You can stretch forth your hand and touch and agree with someone else for healing in your life and for the land.

#71 - Acts 5:16 NIV

Crowds gathered also from the towns around Jerusalem, bringing their sick and those tormented by impure spirits, and all of them were healed.

#72 - Acts 8:7 NIV

…many who were paralyzed or lame were healed.

According to His Word, even the paralyzed can be healed. Nothing is impossible with God.

#73 - Acts 9:34 NIV

"Aeneas," Peter said to him, "Jesus Christ heals you. Get up and roll up your mat." Immediately Aeneas got up.

You may feel like you've been knocked down and can't get up. Perhaps your problems are overwhelming and depression has got you down. It doesn't matter what it is - Jesus can heal you. Get up, roll up your sleeves, hold you head up high and STEP forth and walk in your healing.

#74 - Acts 28:8 NIV

His father was sick in bed, suffering from fever and dysentery. Paul went in to see him and, after prayer, placed his hands on him and healed him.

If you don't have anyone to place their hands on your head, you can do it yourself and you shall be healed.

#75 - James 5:16 NIV

Therefore, confess your sins to each other and pray for each other so that you may be healed. The prayer of a righteous person is powerful and effective.

#76 - 1 Peter 2:24 NIV

"He himself bore our sins" in his body on the cross, so that we might die to sins and live for righteousness; "by his wounds you have been healed."

#77 (3 versions)

3 John 1:2 NIV

Dear friend, I pray that you may enjoy good health and that all may go well with you, even as your soul is getting along well.

3 John 1:2 KJV

Beloved, I wish above all things that thou mayest prosper and be in health, even as thy soul prospers. 3 John 1:2

3 John 1:2 AMP

Beloved, I pray that you may prosper in every way and that your body may keep well, even as I know your soul keeps well and prospers.

This scripture demonstrates how much God loves us. His desire to heal us and for us to prosper and be in good health is a testament to God's divine love. He doesn't want to see anyone perish regardless of some of the past choices and sin. Receive your great health today, receive your prosperity and walk in divine favor and be made whole.

YOUR PERSONAL PRAYER

(Pray Out Loud)

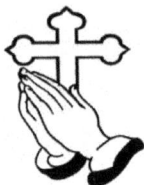

Our Father which art in Heaven, Hallowed, Mighty, Great and Powerful is your name. Let your Kingdom come and let your will be done in my life. Thank you for my daily bread... (the word). Forgive me for all my sins and debts as I forgive those that have sinned against me. Help me when I am tempted and save me from the evil one. For thine is the Kingdom the Power and the Glory, forever in Jesus Name!

Complete your personal prayer that's specific to your situation

Dear God, I need healing in
_____,
I know that you already paid the price and
by your stripes, I am healed. I will not
allow what you did on the cross to be in-
vain, by not receiving your healing virtues.
Therefore, I pray that I am healed.
(Continue writing your personal prayer
request below)

_____

_____

_____

_____

_____

_____

_____

Conclusion

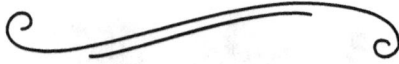

"When he had received the drink, Jesus said, "It is finished." With that, he bowed his head and gave up his spirit" John 19:30 NIV

Three (3) of the most powerful words that seals the deal in any area of life, are "It is FINISHED." When Jesus spoke that out of his mouth, He meant it. Every problem or situation that we may face in our life has already been purchased and paid for. He concluded the matter and redeemed us through His precious blood when He said it was finished. Whether you are experiencing difficulties in your Health, Finance, Faith, or Relationships, it can be RESTORED and you can be

HEALED, because Christ already PAID THE PRICE and by His Stripes you are HEALED!

Appreciation

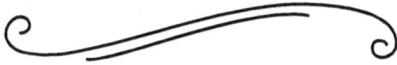

First, I thank God for giving me life, health and strength and the many gifts to be who I am today. I thank Him for all the problems and situations that I went through in the four areas of life. Had I not gone through them, I would not have the ability to write about the journey, the process and how to overcome. Thanks to Jesus Christ for being my savior and to the Holy Spirit for being my guide. Thanks to the most wonderful man on Earth - my husband Kevel A. Anderson, Sr., who loves me with all his heart and gives me the space and time that I need to live out my purpose in life. To our beautiful daughters, Christina and Chassidy and our son A.J. and nephew (like a son), C.J. for their love, laughter and support. To my mom, Sharon and a host of family and friends, thank you! To Latreeta, my friend and prayer partner, who would not stop pushing me to write this book. She wanted to be the first to purchase it. To the staff and friends at Riley Press, Integrity Consulting Enterprise and Kidd Marketing, thank you. To you that have purchased this book - thank you! I pray God's divine healing in any area of your life.

About the Author

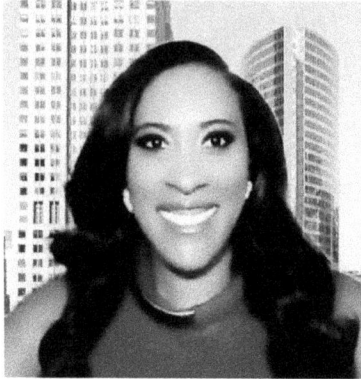

Dr. Carolyn G. Anderson is the FRESH, dynamic and inspirational VOICE that's creating a buzz locally, nationally and internationally. She's a Philanthropist, TV Personality, Wealth Coach, Professor and the author of several books such as LiFE on Purpose, Focus & Get Results, The 10 Laws of LeaderSHIP, Pregnant with a Promise, From the PIT to the PALACE and many more.

One of the nation's leading expert on the art of transformation, she is the Founder and Executive Vice President of Integrity Consulting and Coaching Enterprise (ICE), a corporate coaching, speaking and consulting firm with over

30 years of combined experience in strategic leadership, lean processes, six sigma, visioning, process improvement, coaching, contracting and negotiations, amongst other services.

A trained Army Soldier, Dr. Carolyn knows the discipline and FOCUS needed to hit the TARGET! She utilizes the same skills taught in the military to fight and WIN. She is a trusted voice and a ground-breaking Speaker-preneur. Amongst her many accomplishments and accolades, her all-time favorite role is being a mom and wife. Being a parent is a gift from God. She is purpose driven and lives life fully every day always walking in her divine calling. Learn more about her at www.carolynganderson.com

Connect with us!

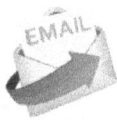

I would like to hear from you and your wonderful testimony of your healing and the difference that this book made on your life. You can email us at admin@carolynganderson.com

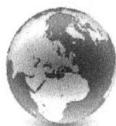

Learn more about other products and services or for booking at www.carolynganderson.com

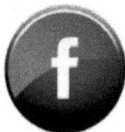

Like our Page www.facebook.com/DrCarolynAnd

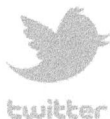

Follow us at: www.twitter.com/DrCarolynAnd

Thank you!

Books by Carolyn G. Anderson

Pregnant with a Promise

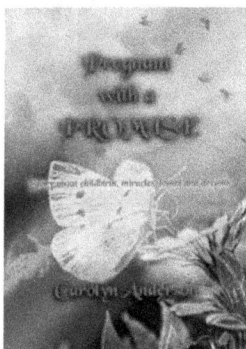

Focus & Get Results

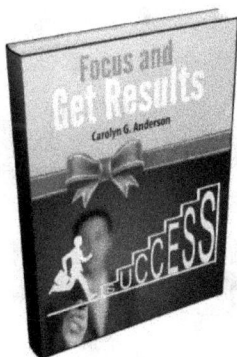

2017 / 5777 – The Year of Victo-ries
#7YearSeries

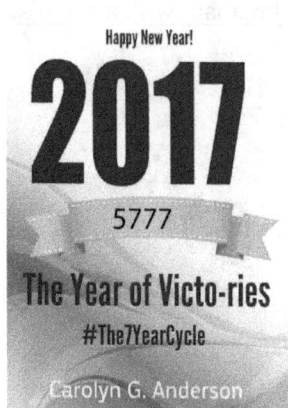

Living a WEALTHY LiFE on Purpose

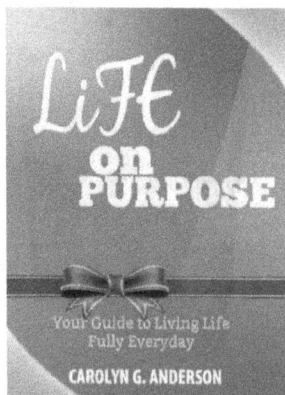

The 10 Laws of Lead-er-SHIP

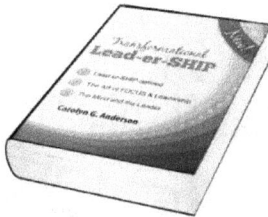

What Happens When the Dream Dies?

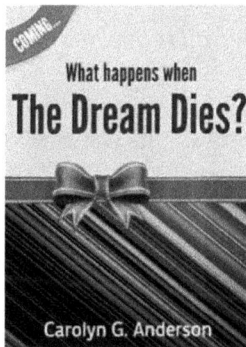

7 Steps to Break-through (Digital/Audio)

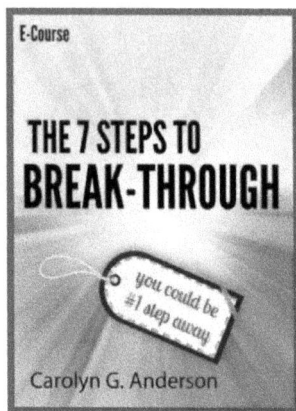

Join our book club at DrCarolynBookClub on Facebook and stay connected with us. Here you can start your own mini-book club and participate with all that Dr. Carolyn is doing. We would be delighted if you're a part of what we're doing.

Notes…………

www.ingramcontent.com/pod-product-compliance
Lightning Source LLC
Chambersburg PA
CBHW070923270326
41927CB00011B/2699

9780996403832